LifeSkills Training

Promoting Health and Personal Development

Student Guide 1

Gilbert J. Botvin, Ph.D.

Professor Emeritus
Weill Cornell Medical College
Cornell University

Princeton Health Press
1.800.293.4969
www.lifeskillstraining.com

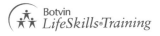
Botvin
LifeSkills®Training

CJK0319

LifeSkills Training Middle School program, Level 1, Student Guide

ISBN: 978-0-9835782-3-9

Acknowledgements

We would like to acknowledge the assistance of the following individuals at National Health Promotion Associates:

Christopher Williams, Ph.D., Senior Vice President
Craig Zettle, Vice President
Kathleen Silloway, Developmental Editor

We would also like to thank our design consultants at Papercut Studio and instructional consultant at Circa Learning, LLC.

Please visit the *LifeSkills Training* Middle School companion website at www.lifeskillstraining.com/msweb

For more information, please visit www.lifeskillstraining.com

Table of Contents

6 Introduction
6 The Importance of LifeSkills
7 The Purpose of This Program
8 Class Material and Practice
8 How the Program Is Organized
9 Ground Rules

10 Self-Image and Self-Improvement
11 Self-Image and How It Develops
12 Worksheet 1: How I See Myself
13 Worksheet 2: Taking Stock
14 Setting and Achieving Personal Goals
15 Worksheet 3: Recording My Progress

16 Making Decisions
17 Deciding Things on Your Own
17 The 3 Cs of Effective Decision-Making
18 Worksheet 4: Everyday Decisions
19 Worksheet 5: Putting the 3 Cs Into Practice
20 Worksheet 6: My Decision-Making Planner

22 Smoking: Myths and Realities
23 Smoking: Myths and Realities
24 Worksheet 7: Who's Using Drugs?
25 Smoking and Your Body
26 Other Ways Smoking Can Hurt You
27 Worksheet 8: My Reasons for Not Smoking

28 Smoking and Biofeedback
29 Immediate Effects of Cigarette Smoking
30 Why Smoking Makes Your Heart Beat Faster
32 How to Take Your Own Pulse
33 Worksheet 9: My Observations
34 Smoking Crossword Clues
35 Smoking Crossword Puzzle

36   Alcohol: Myths and Realities
37   Drinking Fact Sheet
38   Reasons Why Many People Don't Drink
39   Getting a Grip on Reality
40   Worksheet 10: My Reasons for Not Drinking

42   Marijuana: Myths and Realities
43   Marijuana Fact Sheet
44   Worksheet 11: My Reasons for Not Using Marijuana

46   Advertising
47   Common Advertising Techniques
50   Worksheet 12: Practice Analyzing Ads
51   Worksheet 13: Practice Analyzing Tobacco and Alcohol Ads

52   Violence and the Media
52   What Is Violence?
53   Worksheet 14: Watching TV
55   Worksheet 15: Reality Checks

56   Coping with Anxiety
57   How to Decrease Your Anxiety
58   Worksheet 16: Dealing with Anxiety
59   Worksheet 17: Rating How Anxious You Feel

60   Coping with Anger
61   Staying in Control
62   Worksheet 18: What Really Bugs Me

64   Communication Skills
65   Why Communication Skills Are Important
66   Worksheet 19: Looking at a Recent Misunderstanding
67   Communicating Clearly: Skills for Avoiding Misunderstandings
68   Worksheet 20: Practice Applying Communication Skills

70 Social Skills

71 Getting Over Being Shy

73 Tips for Starting a Conversation

75 Worksheet 21: Developing Social Skills Scripts

76 Worksheet 22: Social Activities

78 Assertiveness

79 How to Be More Assertive

80 Worksheet 23: Handling Difficult Situations

81 Refusal Techniques: Ways of Saying "No"

82 Worksheet 24: Assertive Action Plan

83 Worksheet 25: Additional Action Plan

84 Resolving Conflicts

85 Changing You and Me to We

Introduction

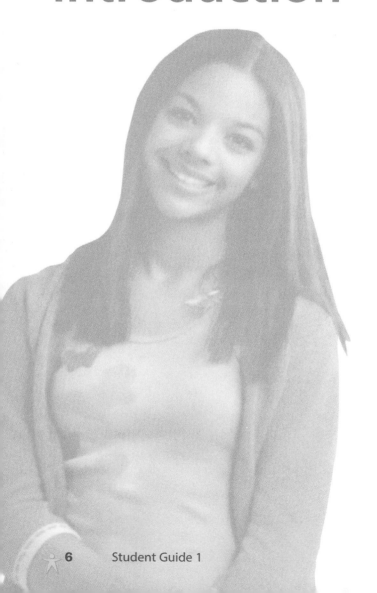

The Importance of LifeSkills

We live in a complex and challenging world. To succeed in this world and effectively deal with the many problems facing us, we require a specific set of skills. We call these skills *life skills*. Surprisingly, these important skills are not usually taught to us in school; they are not usually taught to us at home, in college, or on the job; in fact, they are rarely taught at all. Instead, we are somehow expected to learn the skills we need to live happy, healthy, and successful lives totally on our own.

Although people do learn these life skills on their own, they often learn them in a hit-or-miss way. Unfortunately, many people may go through their entire lives without learning these skills or only partially learning them.

The Purpose of This Program

The *LifeSkills Training* program was developed by psychologist Gilbert J. Botvin, Ph.D., to provide an organized way for students to learn these important skills. Dr. Botvin discovered that students who received this program were not only better prepared to deal with the challenges of life but also less likely to smoke, drink, or use drugs. The *LifeSkills Training* program not only prevents tobacco, alcohol, and drug abuse but also teaches the knowledge and skills necessary to:

- Increase your self-esteem
- Increase your ability to make decisions and solve problems
- Communicate effectively
- Avoid misunderstandings
- Manage anxiety
- Make new friends
- Stand up for your rights
- Say "no" to unfair requests
- Resist advertising pressures
- Resist pressure to use drugs

Class Material and Practice

Your **Student Guide** includes material that your teacher will refer to in class, some general background information, and exercises to be completed at home or in class. These exercises are designed to help you get the most out of the *LifeSkills Training* program; therefore, it is important for you to do them. It is also important for you to practice the skills. It is only by practicing them and applying them to your life every day that you will fully master them.

These exercises are designed to help you learn how to use "life skills." Your **Student Guide** is an important source of information that can be referred to over and over.

How the Program Is Organized

After a general introduction by your teacher, the program starts with information and skills that will help you develop a positive self-image. Next, it focuses on learning how to make decisions without being influenced too much by other people, by advertisements, and by things you see or hear in the media (TV, the Internet, newspapers, movies, etc.). The program also includes material on how to resist pressures to smoke, drink, or use other drugs. The program then focuses on the best ways of dealing with anxiety, communicating with others, and building friendships. It ends by teaching skills for saying "no" to unfair requests and offers to use drugs.

This is a great program which has already helped students just like you. We are confident that you will find it personally valuable and fun.

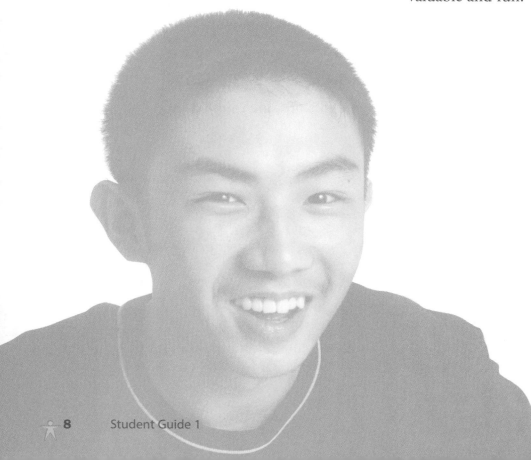

Ground Rules

Here are some basic guidelines for the program.

Program Guidelines

• Only one person talks at a time.

• Everyone should have the opportunity to participate.

• Students are free to express their opinions or participate in group activities without being subjected to criticism.

• Respect your fellow students; listen to them and their ideas.

• Anything discussed in the group remains confidential.

• In the space below, list additional rules suggested by the class:

_____

_____

_____

_____

_____

_____

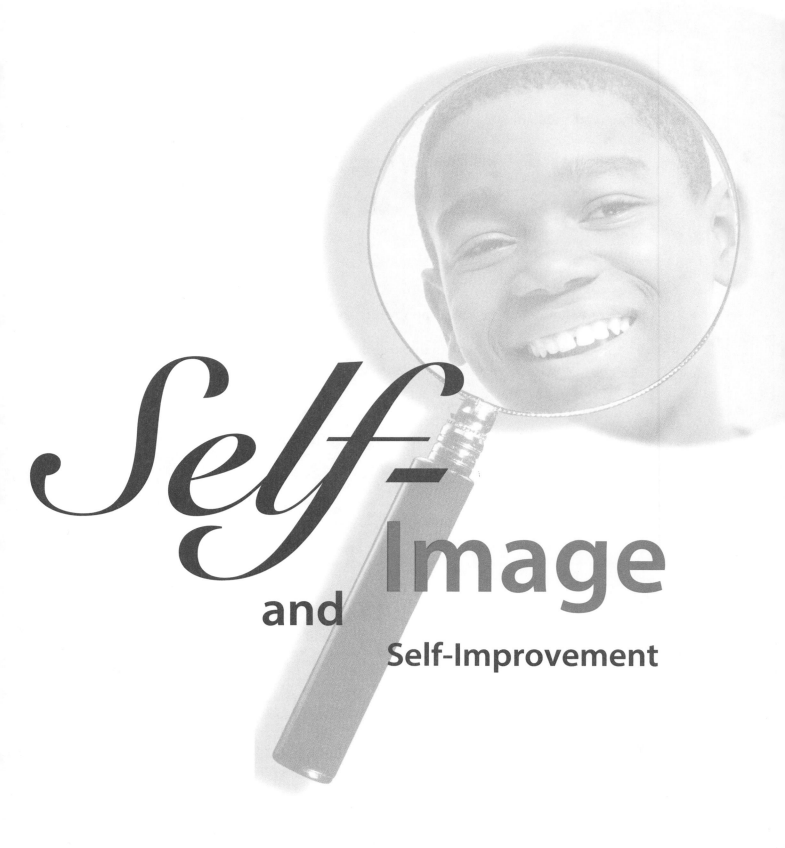

Self-Image and Self-Improvement

Self-Image and How It Develops

What do we mean by the term *self-image*? Self-image is simply how we see ourselves: the mental picture or image we have of ourselves. The way we see ourselves is formed largely by our past experiences (successes and failures). It can also be affected by what people have told us about ourselves. If all your teachers told you that you were smart, you would probably think you were smart! If people told you that you were good at sports and you did well at sports, you would in all likelihood think of yourself as a good athlete. Self-image is generally a reflection of who we are. However, people don't always see themselves as they really are.

How Self-Image Affects Behavior

Why does it matter if we see ourselves accurately? It's important for two reasons. First, how we see ourselves is important because it affects how we behave, what we do, and how well we do it. It also affects how hard we try. For example, people who think they are good at sports or in school will work hard and usually do well. People tend to act like the person they think they are.

A second reason that self-image is important is that it affects how good you feel about yourself. People who feel good about themselves are more confident, more satisfied, more successful, do better in school, and are more popular than people who see themselves in a negative light. People who have a positive self-image are also less likely to smoke, drink, use drugs, or engage in other unhealthy activities.

Improving Your Self and Your Self-Image

Although most of us have a general self-image, it is usually made up of a number of separate self-images relating to ourselves in specific situations. For example, one person may be a good baseball player, a bad swimmer, a good writer, an average math student, etc., all at the same time.

You can do several things to improve your self-image and self-esteem. First, never form a negative image of yourself after one or two bad experiences. Second, take stock. Look at yourself as realistically as possible. Identify your strengths and weaknesses. Third, work on improving areas where you are weak. You can develop a more positive self-image by setting and achieving goals, by deciding what you'd like to change about yourself or what you'd like to accomplish, and then by doing it.

Describe yourself as you are now and as you would like to be, using three adjectives or short phrases for each situation.

How I See Myself

Myself Now

With Friends
1. Weird
2. Bored
3. not lonley

At School
1. Quite
2. Focused
3. Blending in

At Home
1. I Safe more
2. Comfortable
3. weird

In General
1. Happy
2. weird
3. Blending in

Myself as I Would Like to Be

I don't care
I don't care
I don't care

Quite
focused
Blending in

Safe
comfortable
weird

Happy
weird
Blending in

A. List your strengths and weaknesses.

B. List five things about yourself that you would like to change or improve.
   Rate how important it is to you to change each one.

Taking Stock

A. Strengths   **Weaknesses**

1. Greatfull   Shy

2. Smart

3. Kind

4.

5.

B. Things to Change   **Rate Your Desire to Change**

	High	Average	Low
1. Lazyness	☐	☐	☐
2. Shy	☐	☐	☐
3.	☐	☐	☐
4.	☐	☐	☐
5.	☐	☐	☐

Setting and Achieving Personal Goals

How to Set Goals

1. Pick a goal that is **realistic**. Set a long-term goal for yourself that is possible for you to accomplish within a reasonable amount of time (for example, by the end of the semester).

2. Pick a goal that is **manageable**, that you can break down into a series of small short-term steps (or sub-goals). The best way to change a behavior is to do it in small steps.

3. Pick a goal that is **measurable** (for example, how far you jog) so you can tell whether you have achieved it or how much further you have to improve before you do.

4. Pick something that is **meaningful** to you, something that you really want to do rather than something you feel you should do.

Tips for Achieving Your Goals

1. Have a positive attitude. Believe in yourself and your ability to reach the goal that you set for yourself.

2. Don't be afraid to make mistakes. It's all part of learning and making progress toward your goal.

3. If you don't reach a particular goal or sub-goal, don't think of it as a failure. Think of it as a learning experience, as a step toward achieving your goal. Identify what went wrong and correct it.

4. Praise yourself for any progress that you make toward achieving your goal. Tell your friends or parents, and reward yourself.

5. Identify any areas that need further improvement, and work on them with confidence and determination.

6. Use your imagination. Spend some time each day "seeing" yourself achieving your goal.

Write down a goal from the ones you listed on *Worksheet 2, Taking Stock.*

Write a series of sub-goals that lead to it and the dates you expect to reach each one. Allow about a week for reaching each sub-goal.

Check off each sub-goal to show that you have achieved it.

Recording My Progress

Goal

To stop being lazy

Date	Sub-goal	Achieved Sub-goal
March 2	Go on more walks	☐
↓	Play with my dog more	☐
		☐
		☐
		☐
		☐
		☐
		☐
		☐
		☐
		☐
		☐
		☐
		☐

Making Decisions

Deciding Things on Your Own

As you get older, you make more and more decisions on your own. Some of these may be very difficult. To make the best possible decisions, you need to be aware of the people or things around you that can influence your decisions (such as your parents, friends, TV, movies, and advertisements). You also need to learn an organized method for making decisions. Being aware of the factors that might influence your decisions and knowing how to make them can help you to make the best possible decisions for you.

A Simple Method for Making Better Decisions

Most people make all their decisions in the same way, without realizing the difference between simple choices, everyday decisions, and major decisions. Simple choices (whether to eat vanilla or chocolate ice cream) can be decided based on what you like. Other decisions should be made after carefully thinking about the possible consequences, or outcomes, of different decisions. To do this as well as possible and make the best decisions, learn to use the 3-step method described here.

The 3 Cs of Effective Decision-Making

Step 1: Clarify what decision you need to make.

Step 2: Consider the possible alternatives (think about the different things you might decide to do) and the consequences of choosing each alternative; collect any additional information needed. (If you are trying to solve a problem, think up as many solutions as possible.)

Step 3: Choose the best alternative and take the necessary action. Afterwards, think about whether you were satisfied with your decision.

Make a list of the most important decisions you have to make regularly at home, school, or with friends.

Check off whether you make those decisions **On Your Own** or whether you are influenced by others. Check all that apply to each decision.

Everyday Decisions

Decisions	On My Own	Parents	Friends	Teachers	Media
At Home					
1. _____	☐	☐	☐	☐	☐
2. _____	☐	☐	☐	☐	☐
3. _____	☐	☐	☐	☐	☐
4. _____	☐	☐	☐	☐	☐
5. _____	☐	☐	☐	☐	☐
At School					
1. _____	☐	☐	☐	☐	☐
2. _____	☐	☐	☐	☐	☐
3. _____	☐	☐	☐	☐	☐
4. _____	☐	☐	☐	☐	☐
5. _____	☐	☐	☐	☐	☐
With Friends					
1. _____	☐	☐	☐	☐	☐
2. _____	☐	☐	☐	☐	☐
3. _____	☐	☐	☐	☐	☐
4. _____	☐	☐	☐	☐	☐
5. _____	☐	☐	☐	☐	☐

Read each of the situations and (1) **clarify** the problem, (2) list and then **consider** the possible solutions (choices) and their likely consequences, and (3) **choose** the best solution.

Putting the 3 Cs into Practice

Situation 1

Your teacher gave your class a homework assignment that is due the next day and is a large part of your grade for the course. That night there is an important basketball game that all of your friends will be attending. If you go to the basketball game, you won't have time to do your homework, but you know someone who might let you copy her homework.

Clarify the Problem: _____

Consider Possible Solutions   *Possible Consequences*

1. _____   _____

2. _____   _____

3. _____   _____

Choose My Decision: _____

Situation 2

Your friends want to get together at your house after school when no one is home. They want to drink alcohol. You want to be with your friends, but you know your parents will be angry and you'll get in a lot of trouble if your friends drink at your house.

Clarify the Problem: _____

Consider Possible Solutions   *Possible Consequences*

1. _____   _____

2. _____   _____

3. _____   _____

Choose My Decision: _____

Choose two decisions that you have to make now or sometime in the near future. Briefly describe the situation and then (1) **clarify** (identify) the decision to be made or problem to be solved, (2) list and then **consider** the possible solutions (choices) and their likely consequences, and (3) **choose** the best alternative.

My Decision-Making Planner

Situation 1: _____

Problem: _____

Possible Solutions   *Possible Consequences*

1. _____   _____

2. _____   _____

3. _____   _____

My Decision: _____

Situation 2: _____

Problem: _____

Possible Solutions   *Possible Consequences*

1. _____   _____

2. _____   _____

3. _____   _____

My Decision: _____

smoking
Myths and
Realities

THANK YOU
FOR
NOT SMOKING

Smoking: Myths and Realities

▶ **Myth:** Cigarette smoking is not as dangerous as some people say.
Reality: Most health experts agree that cigarette smoking is one of the most serious causes of death and disability in this country.

▶ **Myth:** It's easy to quit smoking.
Reality: Most people are unsuccessful at quitting smoking, even though about 50 percent of all smokers have tried to quit at least once.

▶ **Myth:** Smoking is not something I will have to worry about until I'm old.
Reality: Smoking is something that hurts you now. It hurts you physically by decreasing your ability to perform strenuous activities, elevating carbon monoxide levels and decreasing endurance, staining teeth and fingers, affecting your sense of taste, causing you to smell like smoke, and costing thousands of dollars a year.

▶ **Myth:** Most people smoke cigarettes.
Reality: Relatively few people smoke cigarettes and even fewer are likely to smoke in the future.

▶ **Myth:** Smoking is cool and sophisticated.
Reality: Smoking has become socially unacceptable in most places.

▶ **Myth:** Organic/natural cigarettes and e-cigarettes are healthier than regular ones.
Reality: There are no healthy cigarettes. "Natural" and organic cigarettes still contain nicotine and produce tar and carbon monoxide. E-cigarettes have nicotine and other chemicals that are known to damage people's health. All of these are harmful to the lungs.

Write down the class estimates of the percentage of teenagers who smoke, drink, and use marijuana and other drugs at least once a month. Compare these estimates to recent results of a national survey of 8th, 10th, and 12th graders by The National Institute on Drug Abuse.

Who's Using Drugs?

Substance	Class Estimate	8th Grade (%)	10th Grade (%)	12th Grade (%)
Cigarettes		2.6	4.9	10.5
E-Cigarettes		6.0	10.0	12.0
E-Vaporizers		6.2	11.0	12.5
Smokeless Tobacco		2.5	3.5	6.6
Alcohol		7.3	19.9	33.2
Marijuana/Hashish		5.4	14.0	22.5
Inhalants		1.8	1.0	0.8
Cocaine		0.3	0.4	0.9
Crack		0.2	0.2	0.5
Methamphetamine		0.3	0.2	0.3
Tranquilizers		0.8	1.5	1.9
Hallucinogens (LSD, PCP)		0.6	0.9	1.4
LSD		0.4	0.7	1.0
Heroin		0.2	0.2	0.2
Steroids		0.3	0.3	0.7

Source: Johnston, L.D., O'Malley, P.M., Bachman, J.G. & Schulenberg, J.E. (2016). *Monitoring the Future national survey results on drug use, 1975-2011: Volume I, Secondary school students*. Ann Arbor: Institute for Social Research, The University of Michigan.

Smoking and Your Body

Parts of the Body Affected

Ears

- Affects the nerves and blood vessels in the ears and may lead to hearing loss.

Eyes

- Causes the eyes to become red and may lead to loss of eyesight.

Skin

- Causes the temperature of the skin to drop.

- Causes wrinkles on the face to appear quickly.

Mouth

- Harms the skin covering the lips, tongue, and throat, and may cause food to taste funny.

- Causes bad coughs.

- Causes bad breath and mouth infections.

Lungs

- Makes it harder to breathe normally, which makes it harder to do well in sports.

Heart

- Narrows the blood vessels, making the heart work harder to pump blood through them.

Nose

- Decreases the ability to smell.

Other Ways Smoking Can Hurt You

You probably already know that smoking causes heart disease, cancer, emphysema, and strokes. But it also gives you bad breath, makes your clothes smell, and stains your teeth. Who wants to be friends with someone like that!

Smoking Is Not Popular

Before anyone knew how bad smoking was, many people smoked. Some people even thought it was cool. But that's not true today. Smoking is a thing of the past. It's not cool to smoke these days. The only people who smoke are people who are too hooked to quit.

Recent surveys in the United States indicate that only about 0.6% of eighth graders, 2.2% of tenth graders and 4.2% of twelfth graders smoke cigarettes everyday. Only about 15% of adults (18 years or older) smoke cigarettes. This means that the vast majority of people in the United States do not smoke cigarettes.

Nonsmokers' Rights

People who don't smoke are becoming more assertive regarding their right to breathe clean air and more vocal in their objections to smoking. The main reason nonsmokers have begun standing up for their rights is the growing scientific evidence that secondhand smoke (the smoke from the lighted tip of a cigarette between and from a smoker's exhalation) has a higher concentration of some of the hazardous substances than does mainstream smoke (smoke inhaled by the smoker). Nonsmokers who are in a room with smokers are forced to breathe in these substances and to become involuntary smokers. Involuntary smoking is dangerous, according to the results of recent scientific studies, increasing nonsmokers' risk of getting smoking-related diseases.

List your personal reasons for not wanting to become a cigarette smoker.

My Reasons for Not Smoking

WORKSHEET
8

1. _____

_____

2. _____

_____

3. _____

_____

4. _____

_____

5. _____

_____

6. _____

_____

7. _____

_____

8. _____

_____

9. _____

_____

10. _____

_____

smoking

and
Biofeedback

Immediate Effects of Cigarette Smoking

Smoking Can Affect You Now

Many of the reasons doctors and other health experts give for not smoking have to do with the fact that smoking causes a number of diseases such as heart disease and cancer. These diseases take a long time to develop – some of them as long as 20 or 30 years.

Because it takes so long to experience the symptoms of these diseases, smoking may not seem that bad. In fact, some teenagers may even believe that smoking will not hurt them. They think that adults just talk about the dangers of smoking to scare them. The problem is, even though it may not seem like smoking is hurting your body, by the time you get a disease caused by smoking, it is usually too late.

What many people don't realize is that smoking does have an effect on your body, and that effect is immediate. It occurs within seconds, and can be measured in several different ways. Some of the things that happen after you smoke a cigarette are as follows: your heart beats faster, your hand steadiness decreases, the amount of carbon monoxide in your lungs increases, the temperature of your skin goes down, and the pattern of your brain waves changes.

Heart Rate and Smoking

Heart rate is the number of times that your heart beats each minute. Most people have a heart rate between 60 and 90 beats per minute. Most smokers have faster heart rates than nonsmokers.

Why Smoking Makes Your Heart Beat Faster

Nicotine (a chemical in cigarettes) increases the heart rate by acting on a part of the body called the adrenal glands, found in the kidneys, causing them to release powerful chemicals into the body. These cause the walls of the heart to contract harder and more often. Because nicotine causes an increase in the heart's activity, the heart needs more oxygen. At the same time, carbon monoxide that is inhaled by the smoker from the cigarette reduces the oxygen in the blood, forcing the heart to work harder to get more oxygen to the body.

This means that cigarette and e-cigarette smoking places an extra strain on the heart beyond its normal work. Over time, this may cause such severe damage to the heart that it could stop working. We call this a heart attack.

Interesting Facts

• Physical activity causes the body to need more oxygen, and that makes the heart beat faster.

• People who don't smoke and who exercise regularly (for example, marathon runners) may sometimes have a healthy resting heart rate as low as 30-40 beats per minute.

• Cigarette smoking decreases the delivery of oxygen to the muscles during vigorous exercise, making the effort of the activity more difficult than usual.

• Nicotine increases levels of blood lactate. When exercising, elevated levels of blood lactate can make people feel fatigued or feel like quitting.

• In some people, cigarette smoke can trigger asthma symptoms, making it nearly impossible to exercise until the symptoms subside.

Things to Remember: Heart Rate

- The speed at which your heart beats changes throughout the day. Several things can affect how fast or slow your heart beats. They include physical exercise, emotions, relaxation, and cigarette smoking.

- Smokers have higher heart rates due to the carbon monoxide and nicotine in cigarette smoke.

- People who smoke have a greater risk of heart disease and heart attacks.

Hand Steadiness

Another effect cigarette smoking has on your body is that it decreases hand steadiness. In other words, it causes your hand to shake more. Although this is not always so bad that you can see it, it can be measured using what is called a hand-steadiness or tremor-tension test. It is the nicotine in the cigarette smoke that makes this happen. Nicotine is a stimulant that speeds up your heart and the rate at which you breathe. Most smokers believe that smoking "calms them down," but it really does the opposite.

Things to Remember: Hand Steadiness

- Smoking decreases hand steadiness.

- The nicotine in cigarette smoke acts as a stimulant.

- Rather than "calming you down," smoking makes you more nervous.

How to Take Your Own Pulse

Place the first and second fingers of your right hand on the inside of your left wrist. (The picture demonstrates this.) Next, count the number of thumps (pulsations) that you feel. Use a clock or watch with a second hand so that you can count the number of pulsations you feel in 15 seconds, then multiply that number times 4. This number (pulsations in one minute) is called the *pulse rate*.

Write what you observed in the video.

My Observations

1. _____
_____

2. _____
_____

3. _____
_____

4. _____
_____

5. _____
_____

6. _____
_____

7. _____
_____

8. _____
_____

9. _____
_____

10. _____
_____

Smoking Crossword Clues

ACROSS

2. Instead of calming people down, smoking cigarettes can make them more _____ .

4. After many years of smoking, _____ builds up in smokers' lungs, making them look black.

7. Smokers can develop a hacking _____ .

8. Secondhand _____ can be dangerous to nonsmokers.

9. Regular smokers often develop yellow _____ on their teeth and fingers.

10. Carbon monoxide forces oxygen from the body's _____ blood cells.

11. Cigarette smoking is a main cause of _____ cancer.

12. _____ teenagers are nonsmokers.

13. _____ in tobacco acts as a stimulant.

14. Most regular smokers find that smoking is a difficult _____ to break.

15. _____ is a healthy way to increase the pulse rate.

16. Smoking has become less socially _____ .

DOWN

1. _____ is the colorless and odorless gas in cigarette smoke.

3. Cigarette smoking can make you sick; it is _____ .

5. Smoking cigarettes can make the heart beat _____ .

6. The nicotine in cigarettes is a known _____ .

11. Cigarette smoking shortens this.

14. Smoking increases the chances of having a _____ attack.

Smoking Crossword Puzzle

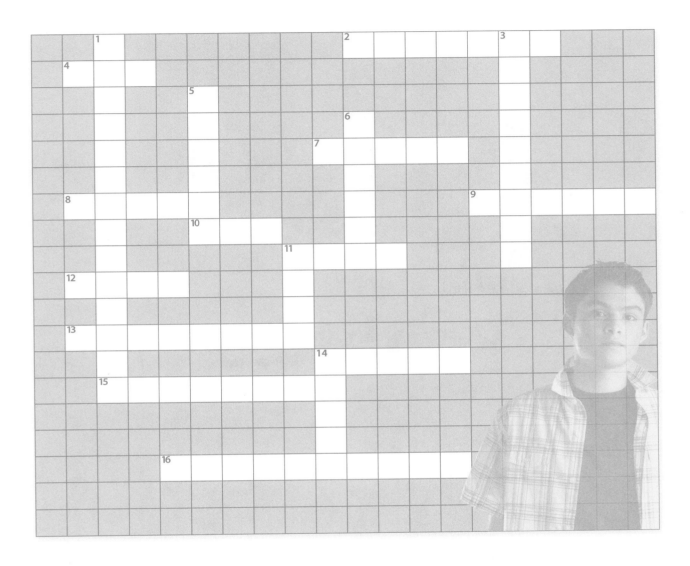

Alcohol

Myths and Realities

Drinking Fact Sheet

What Is Alcohol?

Alcohol is a drug contained in beverages (drinks) such as beer, wine, wine coolers, and liquor. After you drink it, alcohol is absorbed through the walls of the stomach and intestines, directly into the bloodstream. Then it travels through the blood to the brain. Once it reaches the brain, it depresses or slows down the brain's activity.

What Alcohol Does to the Body

A small amount of alcohol:

- Slows down the ability to think clearly and can cause people to make poor decisions.

- Causes people to feel more daring than usual and take risks.

A larger amount of alcohol:

- Slows down other areas of the brain and nervous system.

- Causes dizziness.

- Decreases coordination.

- Decreases reaction time.

- Makes it harder to speak, walk, and stay awake.

- Causes some people to pass out or temporarily lose their memory.

How Alcohol Affects Behavior

In addition to these effects, drinking alcohol also can lead to fighting, arguing, and violence; talking louder than usual; silliness, giddiness, and giggling; and other foolish or obnoxious behavior.

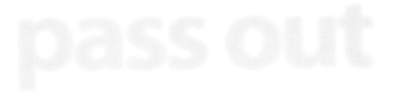

Reasons Why Many People Don't Drink

Many people do not drink or, if they do, drink only once in awhile. Here are some of the reasons people give for not drinking:

- Don't like the taste.

- Don't like getting drunk.

- Don't want to get fat.

- It's against their family values.

- It's against their religious values.

- It's illegal.

- Need to stay in shape for sports.

- Don't want to look stupid.

- Don't want to look foolish.

- Drinking isn't cool.

- Want to stay in control.

- Want to think clearly.

Getting a Grip On Reality

▶ **Myth:** The best way to get "high" is to drink or take drugs.
Reality: Alcohol and drugs produce a temporary "high." With alcohol, the "high" or good feeling it produces goes away after the alcohol wears off. This "up" period is followed by a "down" in which people generally feel tired, ill, depressed, and anxious. The best way to get "high" is the natural way. Some of the ways of achieving a natural "high" are through exercise, sports, dance, music, art, achievement, prayer, meditation, friendship, and love, just to name a few.

▶ **Myth:** It takes a real tough person to hold a lot of alcohol.
Reality: Like other drugs, the more alcohol a person drinks, the more it takes to cause the same effects. This is because people's bodies gradually become tolerant to alcohol. As tolerance increases, so does a person's physical dependence on alcohol and the danger of becoming addicted.

▶ **Myth:** My friends won't want to hang out with me if I don't drink a lot.
Reality: Here's a secret: most people don't really notice how much others are drinking or even what they are drinking.

▶ **Myth:** Drinking beer or wine is OK because there's less alcohol in it.
Reality: A 12 ounce can of beer, 5 ounces of wine, and 1.5 ounces of liquor contain the same amount of alcohol.

▶ **Myth:** Drinking alcohol helps people to sleep better.
Reality: Drinking alcohol can make people sleepy. However, like all depressant drugs, it does not put them into a restful and relaxing state of sleep. The kind of sleep produced by alcohol is not the same as normal sleep. After drinking, people tend to wake up feeling tired, grouchy, and nervous.

List your personal reasons for not drinking alcoholic beverages such as wine, beer, or hard liquor.

My Reasons for Not Drinking

WORKSHEET
10

1. _____
   _____

2. _____
   _____

3. _____
   _____

4. _____
   _____

5. _____
   _____

6. _____
   _____

7. _____
   _____

8. _____
   _____

9. _____
   _____

10. _____
    _____

Notes

Marijuana

Myths and
Realities

Marijuana Fact Sheet

What Is Marijuana?

Marijuana is a dried mixture of leaves, vines, seeds, and stems of a hemp plant called *cannabis sativa*. It is generally used to make homemade "cigarettes" called "joints," which are smoked.

What Does Marijuana Do?

Marijuana affects the person smoking it within minutes. Marijuana produces a "high" or state of intoxication similar to alcohol. Marijuana does a lot more, however, than get people "high." Scientists have discovered that marijuana:

- Causes the heart to beat faster and work harder.

- Raises some people's blood pressure.

- Makes people's hands less steady.

- Causes people to feel sleepy.

- Makes it unsafe to drive a car or operate machines.

- Makes it harder to pay attention.

- Makes it harder to learn new things.

- Makes it harder to remember things.

- Makes some people feel nervous and confused.

- Makes some people feel depressed.

Can Marijuana Do Any Permanent Damage to the Body?

Some of the effects of marijuana can be permanent. Since marijuana smoke contains carbon monoxide and tar, it causes some of the same kinds of health problems as does smoking cigarettes. For example, it can affect people's breathing. And scientists think that, like cigarettes, smoking marijuana regularly for many years may cause certain types of cancer.

List your own personal reasons for not using marijuana.

My Reasons for Not Using Marijuana

1. _____
   _____

2. _____
   _____

3. _____
   _____

4. _____
   _____

5. _____
   _____

6. _____
   _____

7. _____
   _____

8. _____
   _____

9. _____
   _____

10. _____
    _____

Notes

Adver

Common Advertising Techniques

One of the most powerful sources of influence on the decisions we make as consumers comes from advertisements (ads) designed to get us to buy a particular product or service. Advertisers use special methods or techniques to "target" a specific group of people (e.g., parents, teenagers) who are likely to buy the product being advertised. These techniques usually include both a stated message (what the ad actually says) and an implied or hidden message (what is suggested by either the stated message or the overall "look" or "sound" of the ad).

Some common advertising methods or techniques are listed on the next page. If you realize that advertising is intended to get you to buy a product and learn to identify common advertising techniques, you will be better able to make decisions that are right for you instead of being influenced by ads to make decisions that advertisers want you to make.

Identifying Advertising Techniques

Celebrity Endorsement: Has famous or well-known people talk about how great the product is or even claim they use it themselves. Creates the impression that the product must be good if the celebrity uses it.

Bandwagon Appeal: Creates the impression that everybody is using a particular product and that therefore you should, too.

Romance/Sex Appeal: Uses very attractive models in a way that implies that using the product will make you more attractive.

Maturity/Sophistication Appeal: Implies that if you buy a certain product you will be more grown-up, sophisticated, and fashionable.

Fun/Relaxation Appeal: Tries to convince you that buying a product will help you to have more fun or feel more relaxed.

Popularity Appeal: Implies that buying and using a certain product will make you more popular.

Voice of Authority: Uses "experts" such as doctors or scientists (or actors playing the part of experts) to talk about the effectiveness of products such as toothpaste or pain medicine. Advertisers count on consumers believing what experts say about how well the product works.

Scientific Evidence: Presents "facts" and statistics from surveys supporting the effectiveness of particular products. This is often combined with the Voice of Authority technique in an effort to make the ad more convincing.

Advertising

Comparison Tests and Opinion Polls:
Gives the results of consumer opinion polls or "taste tests" involving direct comparisons of similar (competing) products. These ads are intended to show that more people like brand A than brand B, or that product X is stronger, safer, lighter, less expensive, etc., than other similar products.

Demonstrations: Shows how well a product works (usually under the most favorable conditions possible). Some of these demonstrations have been found to be rigged by advertisers to make the product look much better than it really is.

The "Deal" Appeal: Tries to create a sense of urgency and excitement by implying that this is a deal that is too good to pass up. Generally focuses on price and creates a sense of urgency by saying that the deal is only good for a few days and/or that supply is limited.

Write the names of two products or services being advertised, a brief description of the ad, the target market, the stated message(s), the implied or hidden message(s), and the ad technique(s) used to sell these products.

Practice Analyzing Ads

Product Name #1

_____

Description of Ad

_____

_____

Target Market

☐ females   ☐ teens
☐ males   ☐ children
☐ adults   ☐ other:

Stated Message(s)

_____

_____

Implied Message(s)

_____

_____

Technique(s) Used

☐ celebrity
☐ bandwagon
☐ romance/sex appeal
☐ maturity
☐ fun/relaxation
☐ popularity
☐ voice of authority
☐ scientific evidence
☐ comparison test
☐ demonstration
☐ "deal" appeal

Product Name #2

_____

Description of Ad

_____

_____

Target Market

☐ females   ☐ teens
☐ males   ☐ children
☐ adults   ☐ other:

Stated Message(s)

_____

_____

Implied Message(s)

_____

_____

Technique(s) Used

☐ celebrity
☐ bandwagon
☐ romance/sex appeal
☐ maturity
☐ fun/relaxation
☐ popularity
☐ voice of authority
☐ scientific evidence
☐ comparison test
☐ demonstration
☐ "deal" appeal

Write the name of a tobacco and alcohol product being advertised and a brief description of the ad. Identify the target market, the stated message(s), the implied or hidden message(s), and the ad technique(s) used to sell these products.

Practice Analyzing Tobacco and Alcohol Ads

Tobacco Ad

Product Name

_____

Description of Ad

_____
_____

Target Market
- ☐ females   ☐ teens
- ☐ males   ☐ children
- ☐ adults   ☐ other:

Stated Message(s)

_____
_____

Implied Message(s)

_____
_____

Technique(s) Used
- ☐ celebrity
- ☐ bandwagon
- ☐ romance/sex appeal
- ☐ maturity
- ☐ fun/relaxation
- ☐ popularity
- ☐ voice of authority
- ☐ scientific evidence
- ☐ comparison test
- ☐ demonstration
- ☐ "deal" appeal

Alcohol Ad

Product Name

_____

Description of Ad

_____
_____

Target Market
- ☐ females   ☐ teens
- ☐ males   ☐ children
- ☐ adults   ☐ other:

Stated Messages(s)

_____
_____

Implied Message(s)

_____
_____

Technique(s) Used
- ☐ celebrity
- ☐ bandwagon
- ☐ romance/sex appeal
- ☐ maturity
- ☐ fun/relaxation
- ☐ popularity
- ☐ voice of authority
- ☐ scientific evidence
- ☐ comparison test
- ☐ demonstration
- ☐ "deal" appeal

What Is Violence?

Violence is an act or threat that hurts a person or object physically (such as hitting, kicking) or verbally (such as insults, yelling).

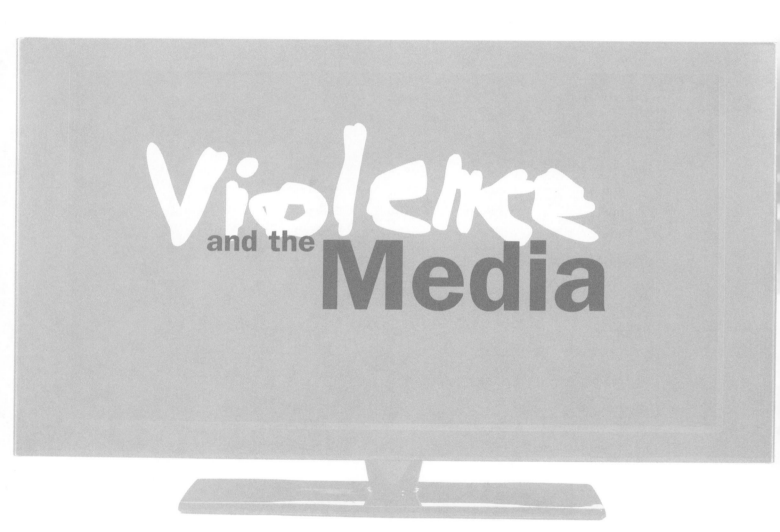

Violence and the Media

A. List the TV shows and movies you watch for a week. Check whether the main characters in each show smoke, drink, use drugs, or act violently.

B. Choose one or two TV shows. List any different violent acts portrayed in each one. Check whether an act shows physical or verbal violence. If it happens more than once, circle the act.

Watching TV

A. Name of Movie or Show	Smoke	Drink	Drug	Violence
_____	☐	☐	☐	☐
_____	☐	☐	☐	☐
_____	☐	☐	☐	☐
_____	☐	☐	☐	☐
_____	☐	☐	☐	☐
_____	☐	☐	☐	☐
_____	☐	☐	☐	☐

B. Name of Show #1

_____

Description of Act	Physical	Verbal
1. _____	☐	☐
2. _____	☐	☐
3. _____	☐	☐
4. _____	☐	☐
5. _____	☐	☐
6. _____	☐	☐
7. _____	☐	☐
8. _____	☐	☐

(continued)

Choose one or two TV shows. List any different violent acts portrayed in each one. Check whether an act is physical or verbal violence. If it happens more than once, circle the act.

Watching TV (Continued)

B. Name of Show #2

_____

Description of Act	Physical	Verbal
1. _____	☐	☐
2. _____	☐	☐
3. _____	☐	☐
4. _____	☐	☐
5. _____	☐	☐
6. _____	☐	☐
7. _____	☐	☐
8. _____	☐	☐

Do a reality check when you watch your favorite movies or TV shows. Here are some questions to ask.

Reality Checks

	Yes	No
1. Is this what happens in real life?	☐	☐
2. Do I agree with this image?	☐	☐
3. Is there a good reason for this violence? Is it trying to make a point, or is it just there to give viewers a safe thrill?	☐	☐

_____

4. What would be the consequences of this violence in real life?

_____

	Yes	No
Are these consequences shown?	☐	☐
5. Are the good guys always right no matter what they do?	☐	☐
6. Are the bad guys shown as deserving what they get, even if it's vigilante, or illegal violence?	☐	☐
7. Is this the best way to resolve this conflict?	☐	☐

8. How else might this conflict be resolved?

_____

_____

_____

_____

Coping
with
Anxiety

How to Decrease Your Anxiety

Deep Breathing

1. Breathe in deeply into your abdomen for a count of 4.

2. Hold it for a count of 4.

3. Breathe out for a count of 4.

4. Repeat 4 or 5 times.

Progressive Muscle Relaxation

1. Sit quietly in a comfortable position with your back straight and feet flat on the floor.

2. Close your eyes.

3. Slowly relax all of the muscles in your body beginning with your toes, working your way up your body to the muscles in your neck and head.

4. Imagine yourself in a quiet, peaceful place (for example, on a beach) feeling relaxed, calm, and without a care in the world.

5. Imagine yourself back in the place where you started the exercise still feeling totally relaxed, peaceful, and calm.

6. Open your eyes and end the exercise.

Practice this exercise as often as possible, at least once a day for about ten minutes each time.

Mental Rehearsal

1. Imagine yourself in an important situation (for example, asking a teacher for more time for a project) feeling completely relaxed and confident.

2. Mentally practice what you will say and/ or do and how you will deal with all the possible things that might happen.

3. Do this over and over again until you begin to feel more relaxed and confident.

Describe two situations that made you feel very anxious, and check off the signs of anxiety that you experienced.

Dealing with Anxiety: Situations That Made Me Feel Anxious

Situation 1

_____

_____

_____

Anxiety Signs (Check off those you felt in Situation 1.)

☐ "Butterflies" in the stomach   ☐ Sweating hands

☐ Rapid heart beat   ☐ Dry mouth

☐ Shaky voice   ☐ Difficulty holding hands still

☐ Muscle tension   ☐ Difficulty concentrating

Situation 2

_____

_____

_____

Anxiety Signs (Check off those you felt in Situation 2.)

☐ "Butterflies" in the stomach   ☐ Sweating hands

☐ Rapid heart beat   ☐ Dry mouth

☐ Shaky voice   ☐ Difficulty holding hands still

☐ Muscle tension   ☐ Difficulty concentrating

Rate how anxious (nervous) you would feel in each situation.

Rating How Anxious You Feel

Situation	High	Average	Low
Taking a test	☐	☐	☐
Giving a report in front of the class	☐	☐	☐
Making a speech in front of a group	☐	☐	☐
Meeting new people	☐	☐	☐
Starting a conversation with someone you just met	☐	☐	☐
Giving someone a compliment	☐	☐	☐
Telling someone that you like them	☐	☐	☐
Asking someone out on a date	☐	☐	☐
Saying "no" when someone offers you beer	☐	☐	☐
Asking someone for a favor	☐	☐	☐
Competing in sports	☐	☐	☐
Singing or playing a musical instrument in front of a group	☐	☐	☐
Saying "no" when someone offers you marijuana	☐	☐	☐
Making an important decision	☐	☐	☐
Saying "no" when someone offers you a cigarette	☐	☐	☐
Saying "no" when someone offers you hard liquor	☐	☐	☐
Telling someone they gave you the wrong change	☐	☐	☐
Returning a product that doesn't work	☐	☐	☐

Coping
with Anger

Staying in Control

The Warning Light

1. Picture a light inside your head. Imagine that it flashes a warning when you need to stop and think before speaking or acting.

2. Remember to check your light whenever you are in a situation that is making you angry.

Counting to Ten (or Higher)

1. Take a deep breath and start counting slowly to yourself.

2. Keep listening to the other person as you count. Don't provoke him or her by revealing what you are doing.

3. Look the other person in the eye.

Self-Statements

Sometimes just telling yourself to stay calm can help keep you calm. Examples of effective self-statements:

- I can resolve this without fighting.

- I can handle this.

- I can stay calm.

- I enjoy feeling calm and in control.

Reframing

Make a mental picture of the situation that's making you angry. Then reframe it – that is, come up with a different way of looking at it. Ask yourself questions like these:

- Is this worth getting angry about?

- Am I sure this person is really out to hurt or insult me?

- Is there another way to get what I want?

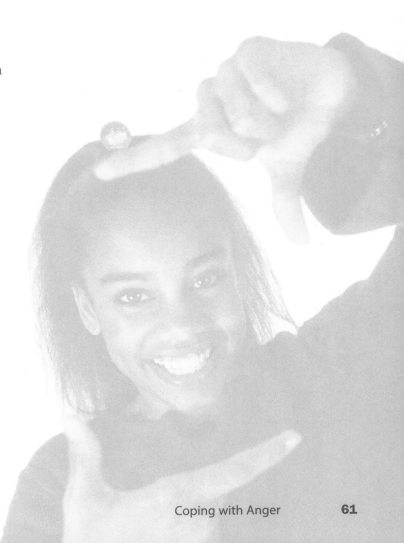

Everyone gets annoyed by one thing or another. List and rate the situations that made you angry this week. Be specific.

What Really Bugs Me

Situation	Rate Your Anger		
	Low	Average	High
1. _____	☐	☐	☐
2. _____	☐	☐	☐
3. _____	☐	☐	☐
4. _____	☐	☐	☐
5. _____	☐	☐	☐
6. _____	☐	☐	☐
7. _____	☐	☐	☐
8. _____	☐	☐	☐
9. _____	☐	☐	☐
10. _____	☐	☐	☐

Communication
Skills

Why Communication Skills Are Important

Since we spend most of our lives with other people, it is important to learn how to get along with others. Learning to communicate effectively can help. Communication is the process by which a person sends a message to another person for the purpose of transmitting information or getting a response. Good communication skills can help us develop satisfying and healthy relationships. Poor communication skills, however, can get in the way of forming and maintaining satisfying relationships and can lead to misunderstandings and bad feelings.

Types of Communication

There are two types or channels of communication: verbal and nonverbal. Verbal communication refers to the specific words that we use as well as the tone and loudness of our voice. Nonverbal communication refers to body language, facial expressions, and gestures. Communication occurs using verbal, nonverbal, or both types of communication. Not sending clear messages using verbal and nonverbal channels of communication or sending verbal and nonverbal messages that don't match can create confusion or result in a misunderstanding.

Describe a recent misunderstanding that you were involved in that resulted from poor communication.

Then identify the specific cause of the misunderstanding and what you think you or the other person could have done to avoid it.

Looking at a Recent Misunderstanding

1. Briefly describe the misunderstanding and who it was with:

_____

_____

_____

_____

2. What was the cause of the misunderstanding? How did the other person feel?

_____

_____

_____

_____

3. How could the misunderstanding have been avoided?

_____

_____

_____

_____

Communicating Clearly: Skills for Avoiding Misunderstandings

A misunderstanding is the result of a failure to communicate clearly. The sender communicates one message, but the receiver hears or sees a different one. Below are some simple ways of communicating clearly and avoiding misunderstandings. Practice these skills and use them as often as possible.

1. **Send the same message on verbal and nonverbal channels.** Make sure what you say matches how you say it. Remember, how you say something is often as important as what you say. Your tone of voice, facial expressions, body position, all send important messages. If you say something with the wrong facial expression, the person hearing you will be confused. For example, if you say you're mad but smile when you say it, the person you're talking to won't think you are serious.

2. **Be specific.** Say exactly what you mean. Unless you are specific, the other person may have to guess what you mean. That can lead to misunderstandings. For example, instead of saying, "I'll see you Saturday afternoon," give a specific time and place ("I'll come over to your house on Saturday at 1 o'clock").

3. **Ask questions.** You can do this whether you are sending or receiving a message. Asking questions works well when explaining how to do something. And if someone tells you something that isn't clear, you can ask that person questions as a way of getting more specific information. For example, "I don't understand, can you explain that again?"

4. **Paraphrase.** Paraphrasing is repeating what someone else said by using your own words. If you tell somebody something and you want to make sure they understand, ask them to paraphrase it. If somebody tells you something and you want to make sure that you have understood it correctly, then you can repeat it back to them. For example, you can say, "OK, let me make sure I understand what you mean." Then say what the person told you.

Read each situation and check off the communication skill or skills that could have been used to avoid the misunderstanding or to clearly communicate the message.

Practice Applying Communication Skills

Situation 1

Andrew arranged to meet a friend at the movies on Friday night at 7 o'clock. That Friday night, Andrew waited and waited for his friend to show up. He concluded that his friend had forgotten or just not bothered to meet him. Meanwhile, his friend was waiting for him at the other movie theater in town, feeling disappointed that Andrew had not shown up or even called to say he wasn't coming.

☐ Send same verbal/nonverbal message   ☐ Be specific

☐ Repeat message back to sender   ☐ Ask questions

Situation 2

Melissa spent the evening baby-sitting for her new neighbor's three children. It had not gone well. The children had not listened to her, and even locked her out of the house for 15 minutes in the cold! She felt very angry. When her neighbors returned she told them about their children's behavior while smiling and laughing about their antics. The children were promised a trip to the toy store the following day for being so good.

☐ Send same verbal/nonverbal message   ☐ Be specific

☐ Repeat message back to sender   ☐ Ask questions

Situation 3

It was an important field hockey game for Carol's team. They were not having a good season. Their coach had worked hard to come up with an effective game plan that would give them a chance to win. Right before the game everyone met to receive specific instructions for their playing position. Carol really didn't understand her instructions very well. During the game she totally messed up and her team lost.

☐ Send same verbal/nonverbal message   ☐ Be specific

☐ Repeat message back to sender   ☐ Ask questions

Notes

social Skills

Getting Over Being Shy

Many people, even famous TV and movie personalities, can be shy and feel uncomfortable in social situations. However, you can learn to be more comfortable in social situations by learning how to deal with anxiety and nervousness and by improving your social skills in social situations. Below are some ideas.

• **Learn to act:** You can learn new social skills and become more self-confident by "playing" a social situation as if you were an actor acting out a specific role.

• **Start small:** Begin by practicing on easy situations, gradually working up to more difficult ones.

• **Prepare yourself:** Write out a brief script and rehearse it at home; watch yourself in the mirror and listen to your voice. This is what actors in plays and movies do.

Saying Hello

Another way to get over being shy is to practice saying hello to people. Below are some common greetings.

• "Hello" or "Hi."

• "How's it going?"

• "Good to see you."

• "Have a good (nice) day."

• Gestures (a nod, smile or wave).

Get in the habit of saying hello to people. The more people you say hello to, the more people who will say hello to you. Most people are shy. You can help them by being the first to say hello.

Meeting New People

Try to meet a lot of new people. Begin a conversation (for example, while standing in line in the lunchroom, at a school sporting event, etc.). Start the conversation with something you think you might have in common. Again, asking questions is an effective method. Below are some examples.

"What are you going to get for lunch today?"

"Is that a good book? What's it about?"

"That's a nice jacket. Where did you get it?"

"Did you see the game last night? Who won?"

Is that a good book?

What's it about?

Who won?

I li

Giving Compliments

An easy way to start conversations and help others feel good is to give a compliment. You can compliment people by looking at:

- What they are wearing
  (e.g., "I like your shirt.")

- How they look
  (e.g., "Your hair looks great.")

- Something they do well
  (e.g., "You're really good at sports.")

- Their personality
  (e.g., "You've got a good sense of humor.")

- Other personal features
  (e.g., "You've got a nice smile.")

Tips for Starting a Conversation

Here are some ideas for starting a conversation with someone you don't know, for example, at a party or dance.

- Pick someone who looks like they would be easy to talk to (a person who seems friendly, is smiling at you, is sitting alone, or is just walking around).

- Introduce yourself. "Hello (Hi), my name is..." Ask each other where you live, what activities you like (e.g., hobbies, sports, etc.).

- Give a compliment and then ask a question. "You were great in the school play. Do you take acting lessons?"

- Ask for or offer help (e.g., help with a package, lending books or pencils, directions, etc.).

- If you can't think of anything to say, you can use such common but very good starters concerning the weather ("The weather has really been great lately") or personal identity ("Are you from around here?" or "Where do you go to school?").

your shirt.

Where did you get it?

Keeping a Conversation Going

Once you begin a conversation, there are several things that you can do to keep things going.

1. Ask questions.
2. Tell a story about yourself.
3. Get the other person talking about him or herself.
4. Let the other person know you are interested in what they are saying.
5. Be happy and "up."
6. Be an active listener. Show that you are listening by using:
   - Verbal cues ("yes," "uh-huh," "I see," "that's really interesting").
   - Nonverbal cues (leaning forward, sitting up, nodding your head, using eye contact).

Ending a Conversation

How you end a conversation can make your next meeting with that person either easier or harder.

1. The ending should be as smooth and natural as possible.
2. Don't cut the other person off in the middle of a sentence. Try to find a natural place to stop.
3. Nonverbal cues can be used to indicate that you want to end the conversation such as breaking eye contact, moving toward the exit, smiling, shaking hands, etc.
4. Be sure the person knows:
   - You are about to leave (end the conversation).
   - You've enjoyed the conversation (or being with the other person).
   - You hope that you will meet (or see each other) again soon.

Develop social skills "scripts." Write down four compliments you could give, four ways of starting a conversation, and four things you could talk about.

Developing Social Skills Scripts

Compliments

1. _____
2. _____
3. _____
4. _____

Conversation Starters

1. _____
2. _____
3. _____
4. _____

Keeping Conversations Going: Things to Talk About

1. _____
2. _____
3. _____
4. _____

Think about the characteristics of people you like to be with and activities you enjoy. Use that information to answer these questions.

Social Activities

1. Describe the kind of person who you would want as a friend – someone you would want to hang out with.

_____

_____

_____

_____

2. List some social activities that you think might be fun to do with others.

_____

_____

_____

_____

3. Describe an approach that you think might work when you're asking if someone wants to get together to do an activity.

_____

_____

_____

Notes

Assertiveness

How to Be More Assertive

Saying "No"

1. **State your position.** Tell the other person how you feel about something, or give your answer to a request that you do something (e.g., "No, you can't borrow my book"). Speak with a strong, confident tone of voice.

2. **State your reason.** Tell the other person the reason for your position, request, or feelings (e.g., "I need to use it myself" or "I already promised that someone else could use it").

3. **Be understanding (if appropriate).** Let the other person know that you understand their point of view, request, or feelings (e.g., "I know you really need to use it, and I wish there was something I could do to help").

Making Requests or Asserting Rights

1. Tell the other person the problem or situation to be changed.

2. Say how you might change the situation or solve the problem. Inform the other person what you would like them to do or what you think (asserting rights), or ask for a favor.

How to Say It

Following these tips will help you be more assertive by using the right nonverbal skills.

1. **Eye Contact:** Look directly into the person's eyes. Don't look away from the person you are talking to or down at the floor.

2. **Facial Expression:** Be certain that your facial expressions match what you are saying (for example, don't smile while telling someone you're angry).

3. **Body position/posture:** Face the person to whom you are speaking, and stand up straight. Slouching will make the person think you don't believe what you're saying.

4. **Distance:** Stand a comfortable distance from the person you are talking with (generally about three feet).

A. Describe a common situation where you have trouble being assertive.
B. List the reason(s) why you don't stand up for your rights or express your true feelings to your friends.
C. Now imagine you are being pressured to smoke cigarettes by friends or classmates. Describe the situation and how you would handle it.

Handling Difficult Situations

A. Situation

B. Reasons Why

C. Describe the situation.

How I would handle it

Refusal Techniques: Ways of Saying "No"

Simple No: "No." or "No, thanks."

Tell It Like It Is: "No, thanks. I don't smoke."

Give an Excuse: "No, thanks. I'm in a hurry right now. I've got to go."

The Big Stall: "No, thanks. Maybe later."

Change the Subject: Say "no" and start talking about something else.

"No, thanks. Hey, did you see the game last night?"

Broken Record: Repeat "no" over and over, or do variations on your "no" response.

"No, thanks."

"No."

"No. I'm not interested."

Walk Away: Say "no" and walk away.

The Cold Shoulder: Ignore the other person.

Avoiding the Situation: Stay away from any situation where you are likely to be pressured to smoke.

Here are some common situations that teenagers find themselves in. How would you handle them? What would you say or do?

Assertive Action Plan

Situation	Your Response
1. You are standing on a long lunch line. Someone cuts ahead of you in line.	_____
2. You are riding a train where smoking is not allowed. The person next to you lights up an e-cigarette.	_____
3. You are in a friend's house and they're drinking beer. Your friends offer you some. You don't want any.	_____
4. Your friend wants to borrow your MP3 player. You don't want to lend it to your friend since you're afraid it will get broken.	_____
5. You're at a party where marijuana is being smoked. You do not want to smoke. Someone passes you a joint.	_____

Describe situations that you think you may have to deal with by being assertive. Write down how you plan to handle them.

Additional Action Plan

Situation	Your Response
1. _____	_____
_____	_____
_____	_____
2. _____	_____
_____	_____
_____	_____
3. _____	_____
_____	_____
_____	_____
4. _____	_____
_____	_____
_____	_____
5. _____	_____
_____	_____
_____	_____

Resolving
Conflicts

Changing You and Me to We

1. Stay Cool

- Take a deep breath.
- Count to ten (or twenty).
- Tell yourself, "I'm too cool to get angry."

  "I feel good when I stay in control."

  "I don't need to fight."

2. Cool Off the Other Person

- Say: "This isn't worth fighting over."

  or "I have nothing against you, and I don't want to fight."

- Use your sense of humor to help the other person lighten up.

3. Listen to the Other Person

- Look him or her in the eye, nod, and say, "I see."
- Restate what is said, then ask, "Is that right?"
- Maintain a respectful distance from the other person. Keep your tone of voice even.

4. Stand Up for Yourself

- Use "I" statements to state your position and tell how you think and feel.
- Give reasons for why you feel as you do.
- Stand tall.
- Speak with confidence.

5. Show Respect

- Don't say what's wrong with the other person.
- Say: "I see where you're coming from."

  or, "I understand why you might feel that way."

- Agree where you can.
- If you've done something wrong, apologize.

6. Solve the Problem

- Suggest a compromise.
- Ask the other person to suggest a compromise.
- Consider other possible solutions.
- Ask problem-solving questions:
  – Why?
  – Why not?
  – What if?
- Consider the possible consequences of each solution.

Notes

Notes

Notes